The skillfully rendered dramatic monologues of Karen Kotrba's *She Who is Like a Mare* document the remarkable history of the Frontier Nursing Service in eastern Kentucky in the early twentieth century. Through the imagined voices of the founder, Mary Breckinridge, and the nurse-midwives she trained to travel the back roads of Kentucky on horseback, Kotrba brings a whole community to life. With a sure command of the multiple tones and mixed dictions of the region, she gives voice to a wide range of characters: the local citizens who are protective of their mountain women who have always "birthed the babies"; the physicians who want to replace any kind of midwifery with the new medical field of obstetrics; the fathers who ride out in fierce storms to bring help to their wives in labor; and the mothers, the children, and even one amazing poem in the voice of a horse. With this book, Karen Kotrba joins the company of our great documentary poets: Stephen Vincent Benet, Carl Sandburg, the Muriel Rukeyser of *U.S. 1*, and West Virginia poet Louise McNeill. She has brought to light a little known piece of women's history—a story of cunning, courage, and caring—and has done so with unforgettable imagery, beautiful music, and love. This is a book I want to keep near me and reread, to remind myself of what is still *possible* in poetry and in our lives.

—Maggie Anderson, author of *Windfall: New and Selected Poems*

She Who Is Like a Mare
Poems of Mary Breckinridge and the Frontier Nursing Service

Karen Kotrba

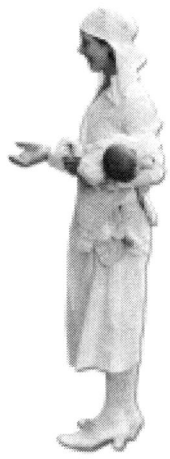

Appalachian Writing Series
Bottom Dog Press
Huron, Ohio

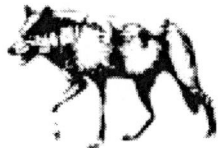

© 2012 Karen Kotrba
& Bottom Dog Press
ISBN 978-1-933964-62-1
Bottom Dog Publishing
PO Box 425
Huron, Ohio 44839
http://smithdocs.net
e-mail: Lsmithdog@smithdocs.net

CREDITS:

General Editor: Larry Smith
Layout & Design: Susanna Sharp-Schwacke
Cover Design: Susanna Sharp-Schwacke and Larry Smith
Author's Photo by Patti Swartz.
Cover Photo from University of Louisville, Kentucky.
Photos from the Caulfield & Shook Collection, Special Collection Library, University of Louisville, Kentucky, and from the Frontier Nursing University.

ACKNOWLEDGEMENTS:

Many people helped this manuscript along the way. I wish to thank the following for their wise counsel and support: Patricia Stout, Jan C. Snow, Patti Swartz, Roxanne Burns, Maggie Anderson, Craig Paulenich, Will Greenway, Mary Biddinger, Lonnis Kirsher, and the Smart Mouthy Women.

Table of Contents

PREFACE
INTRODUCTION
    She Who is Like a Mare..17
    Frontier, Defined..19
    Photograph, Date Unknown..21
SECTION ONE: BEGIN SMALL
    Mary Breckinridge on Grief..25
    A Mountain Doctor Muses..26
    Mary Breckinridge on the Strength of Saplings...........................27
    Local Woman: On Saddlebag Women..28
    Mary Breckinridge Speaks of Burdens...29
    Thus Sayeth the Expert: Dr. Josiah M. Slemons Weighs In on
        the Curse of Eve...31
    Local Woman: Knots..32
    Lady Helen MacKenzie: Scotland Comes to Kentucky...............33
    Thus Sayeth the Expert: Dr. DeLee Calls for the End to
        Midwifery...36
    Gwen's Highland Farewell..38
    Gwen's Journey to Lenore..39
    Kate Meditates on Hills Like Domed Temples.............................40
    A Memo From Mary Breckinridge: This is to Inform You
        That...41
    Lenore Grumbles About Uniformity..42
    Thus Sayeth the Expert: Nurse Scovil Speaks to Prospective
        Mothers..43

SECTION TWO: TAKE ROOT
    Mary Breckinridge Explains Mountain Medicine........................47
    Kate Sees a Haint..48
    Lay of the Land: Sarah's Stall Mucking Song...............................49
    Annie, 7, Skips to the Clinic...50
    Horse Trading: Sales Pitch...51
    Sarah Explains Mountain Etiquette...52
    Mary Breckinridge Calls for Stories...53
    Nancy Tries to Tell It..54
    Sarah's Letter Home: Tower to Tank and Across the Creek.........55
    Horse Trading: Mary Returns a Horse...56
    Kate's Lament...57
    Sarah's Journal: Keening...58
    Horse Trading: Mary Keeps a Horse..59
    Sarah's Letter Home: A Cabin in Arles..60
    Horse Trading: Gift Horse..62

  Kate's Case of Mountainitus..63
  Sarah's Journal: Fecundity..64

Section Three: Grow
  Frontier Nursing Service Bulletin: Will You Fill Their
    Saddlebags..69
  Hyden Man Peruses the Sunday Paper...70
  Annie, 9, Takes a Stand..71
  The Moon Man Speaks..72
  Nancy and the Moon Man..74
  Miss Marvin Makes a Movie: Marvin in the River.........................76
  Lenore at the Brink..77
  Nancy Describes the Topography..78
  Mary Breckinridge Contemplates One Bright Star.......................79
  Lenore Encounters Poetry...80
  Rose: Dead Tired...81
  Tom's Vow...82
  Miss Marvin Makes a Movie: *The Forgotten Frontier*...................83
  Raven Speaks...84
  Sarah Speaks of New Troubles..85
  Miss Marvin Makes a Movie: An Evening of Hoopla.....................86
  Sarah's Letter Home: New Moon...87
  Mary Breckinridge Puts It All in Perspective................................88

Epilogue
  Vespers at Wendover..91

About the Author...93

For Agnes, Annie, and remarkable women everywhere.

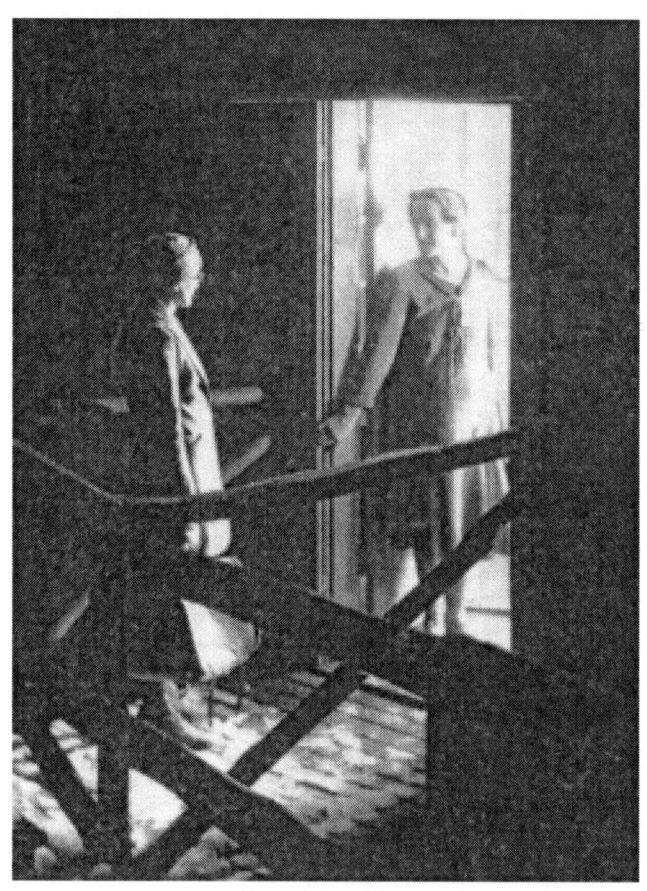

Night Call
(Courtesy of FNU)

Preface

Women. Horses. Babies. Mountains. Eastern Kentucky in the early twentieth century. What I first heard about the Frontier Nursing Service (FNS) seemed romantic: nurse-midwives on horseback, riding cabin to cabin through a rugged mountain landscape, delivering babies and providing other needed medical care. As I explored the subject further, however, I realized the nurses' work was arduous. They used mountain trails and creek beds for roadways, forded rushing waters after spring rains, and delicately crossed the ice in winter. *If the father can get to you*, the rule was, *you are obliged to go with him*. Long days spent in the saddle to get to patients were followed by evenings documenting the day's activities.

The Frontier Nursing Service was founded in 1925 by Mary Breckinridge. *Southern* and *aristocratic* are adjectives often used to describe her background. Her great grandfather was Thomas Jefferson's attorney general. Her grandfather was a U.S. Senator who became James Buchanan's vice president; during the Civil War he was a Confederate general and the Confederacy's last Secretary of War. Mary's cousin, Sophonisba Breckinridge, was a reformer and pioneer in the new field of social work. And Mary's father, Clifton Breckinridge, served in the U.S. House of Representatives. When President Grover Cleveland appointed him ambassador to Russia, Mary spent part of her girlhood in St. Petersburg, Russia and in a girls' school in Switzerland.

In Mary's autobiography, *Wide Neighborhoods*, she credits her great aunt with awakening her interest in Kentucky. The aunt was, in Mary's words "a wealthy and charitable woman" who donated money to support young people of her home state through high school and college. Mary later used money which she inherited from her great aunt to start the Frontier Nursing Service.

After an early marriage ended in widowhood, Mary trained as a nurse from 1907-1910, a career she left after she remarried. By 1918 Mary suffered devastating losses: a daughter born prematurely lived only six hours, and her son, "Breckie," died from a sudden illness two weeks after his fourth birthday. Her second marriage ended in divorce.

In 1918, a few months after her son's death, she volunteered to work with the American Committee for Devastated France. There she encountered a rural population traumatized by war: villagers lacking necessities, fields with mines in them, and few nurses and fewer doctors.

Mary stayed in France until 1921 helping to reinstate medical services. While there she was impressed by the couriers, girl chauffeurs who volunteered to truck supplies into the villages. Meeting British nurse-midwives made an impact on her as well. At that time, French midwives were not nurses and in America, nurses were not midwives. Seeing the wisdom of combining the two professions, Mary went to England to become a midwife.

After her training Mary traveled the Scottish Highlands and Hebrides Islands to observe nurse-midwives making their rounds by bicycle or on foot. Determined to implement a similar model in a remote area of the United States, Breckinridge decided that eastern Kentucky was the logical location. Before the FNS was in operation, most babies in Appalachia and other impoverished or isolated parts of America were delivered by granny midwives, local women who lacked formal medical training but provided the best care they could. Infant and maternal mortality rates were high.

Breckinridge turned her grief over the deaths of her children and her family legacy of public service into a passion for improving the survival rate of newborns and their mothers in Kentucky's mountains. She took special measures to avoid appearing as "Lady Bountiful" come to save the mountaineers. She traveled throughout the region on horseback, meeting and listening to as many people as she could, including the granny midwives.

In the years that followed, Mary organized a local committee of advisors, purchased land on the middle fork of the Kentucky River, and constructed a two-story log building to serve as FNS headquarters, its first clinic, and her home. She named it Wendover. Mary soon spearheaded the construction of a twelve-bed hospital in nearby Hyden. (Sir Leslie MacKenzie, Scotland's chief medical officer, who had welcomed Mary when she observed Highland nurses, spoke at the hospital's dedication ceremony.) When Mary added six outpost clinics in Leslie County and parts of Clay and Perry counties, FNS nurse-midwives were able to care for families in an area of more than 600 square miles. Care for the horses as well as delivery of supplies and messages between the FNS facilities was performed by the couriers, who were young female volunteers.

In 1939, when most of the nurse-midwives returned to the United Kingdom for the war effort and it became impossible to send American nurses overseas for training, Mary founded the Frontier Graduate School of Midwifery.

Much of what has been written about the FNS stresses the organization's accomplishments, but what of the day-to-day lives of the individuals involved? The poems that follow are my attempt to imaginatively flesh out what is documented about the lives of these women. Two of the figures are drawn from actual women: Mary herself and her cousin Mary Marvin Breckinridge (who was called by her middle name.) "Nancy," an Irish nurse-midwife is loosely based on Nancy O'Driscoll, who died while in service to the FNS. Others are my inventions. Among them are Lenore, a Scottish nurse-midwife, and Sarah, a courier. I derived ideas for the poems from published materials about the FNS, including Mary's autobiography *Wide Neighborhoods*, and items at the FNS archives at the University of Kentucky in Lexington.

Pregnancy guidebooks for middle-class women provided cultural context, and my observations at Wendover and Hyden also informed the poems. Although the FNS history spans more than eighty-five years, the early years (1925-1935) most inspired the poems.

By Mary's death in 1965, the FNS had delivered 14,500 babies and cared for more than 57,000 patients. Mary Breckinridge and the FNS occupy a unique place in both Appalachian history and the history of American nursing. Today Frontier Nursing University continues the FNS mission, providing advanced degrees in midwifery and family nursing "from the birthplace of nurse-midwifery and family nursing in America."

Wendover is now a bed and breakfast. Staying there a couple of nights, one imagines hearing the couriers bustling in the kitchen as they prepare afternoon tea for the nurse-midwives. Sleep in Mary's bedroom soothed by a lullaby of night insects outside her window. Perhaps in your dreams you will see a nurse heave a saddlebag onto her horse and set off for a delivery. You will awaken awed by Mary Breckinridge and the courage of the women who carry her vision forward.

—Karen Kotrba, August 2012

"I learned that it is wise to begin small, take root, and then grow."

Mary Breckinridge
Wide Neighborhoods:
The Story of the Frontier Nursing Service

INTRODUCTION

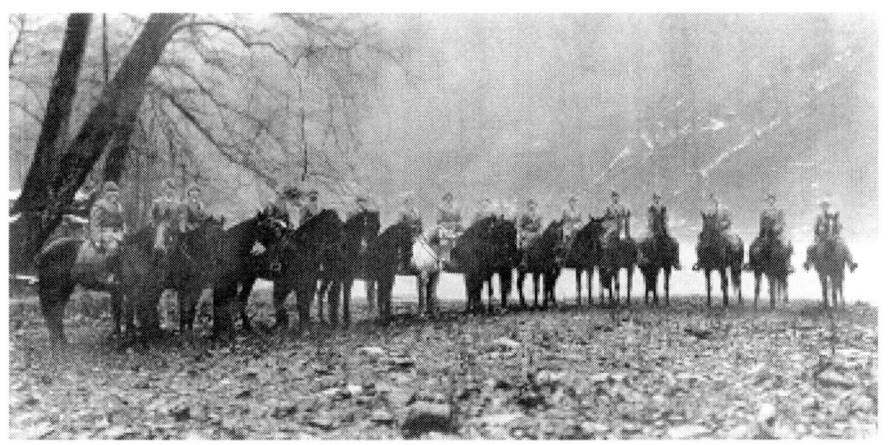

Line Up
(Courtesy of FNU)

SHE WHO IS LIKE A MARE

Epona rides the womansaddle.
>She holds a horn filled with wheat
in her left hand, while her right
strokes the mane. A foal follows.

Sometimes
>Epona is enthroned, flanked
by horses who dine on apples
warm from the bowl of her lap.

From Gaul
>legions carried the mare goddess
to Rome where they boxed her in
stables, draped her with roses.

Only the Celts
>gave her sway over rivers, streams,
begged blessings for crossings
of both the rider and the steed.

Frontier, Defined

Frontier (*n.*) 1. A vast, largely unknown space of land just beyond the known: As in, in May 1932 Sarah arrived at this *frontier* to serve four months as a volunteer courier.

2. The area between civilization and a more natural, unrefined country; a place on the edge; a dreamscape of risk and adventure.

3. An ill-defined place, wild, potentially dangerous though not necessarily including cowboys, Indian raids, cattle drives, and shootouts: Sarah's future was a *frontier* she hardly dared to ponder.

4. A place without roads or plumbing.

5. A wilderness large enough to feel small in, unlike the comfortable containment of the train Sarah takes to Hazard; also, a place in which Sarah can grow (in ways as yet undefined).

6. A euphemism that daubs a romantic glow upon a region forgotten, neglected: Because no one else will, nurse-midwives provide care for mothers and children across 52 square miles of Appalachian *frontier*.

7. A new sort of knowledge, the result of innovation, often expressed in the plural. Working at the *frontiers* of medicine, Mary Breckenridge decentralized medical care by establishing clinics in the mountains of Eastern Kentucky.

(*adj.*) 1. Of, on, near or in regard to a frontier: To improve the health of mothers and babies, Mary Breckenridge founded the *Frontier* Nursing Service in 1925.

Photograph, Date Unknown

What can we know about these women? Sixteen of them, all on horseback,
panoramed in a wobbly arc shallower than a horseshoe. The photographer–
assumed male, given the era–positions the camera left of center.

This makes Mary, first in line, loom closest. He steps back,
to reveal a slim foreground of fallen leaves, a slice of sky and
bare branches. Do the horses jostle each other as riders crowd into place?

Do the novices grin apologies for the difficulties of lining up just so?
Riders sit erect. Mary has lectured on the fundamentals of posture,
but only she appears at ease, loose arms, not clutching reins or saddle horn.

From this far back the others are as anonymous as soldiers on the field, alike
in blue uniforms, brimless hats. There is no knowing which are the Scottish nurses,
lured by tales of horses and dogs and life in the mountains. No telling which

is the Irish girl who will die, appendix too late removed, her horse led riderless
to a funeral down a trail. From here the nurses' expressions are lost but Mary
looks pleased. Her plan is working. Even now, couriers in Wendover are steeping tea.

Section One

Begin Small

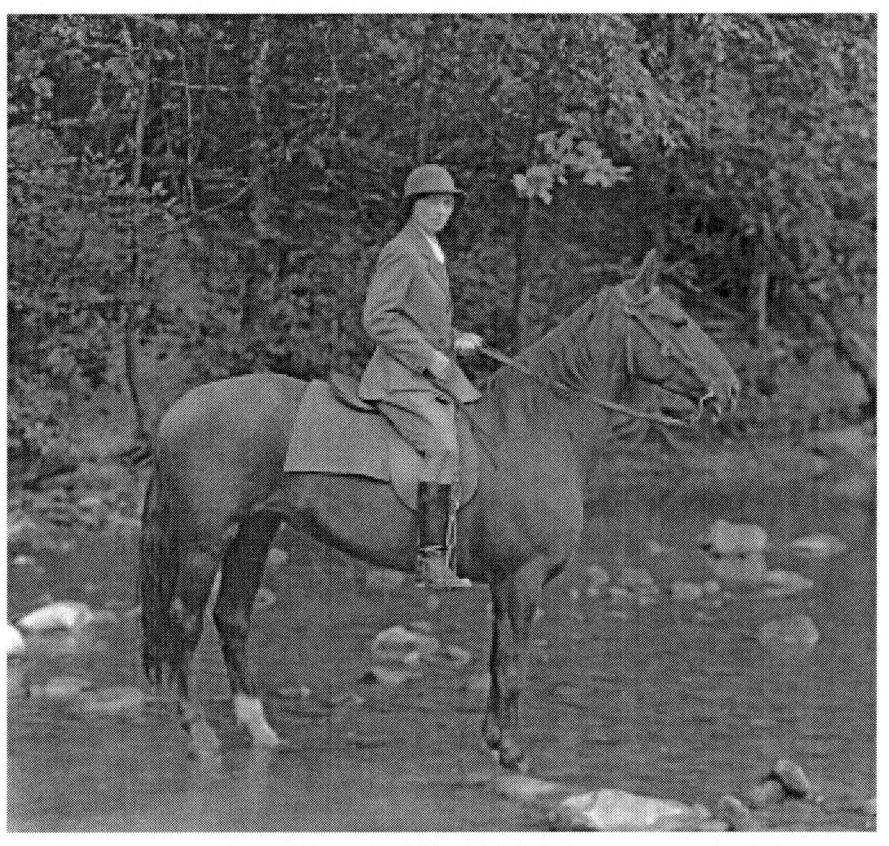

Nurse fording a stream on horseback, Wendover, Kentucky, 1931.
(Courtesy University of Louisville)

Mary Breckinridge on Grief

What happens when your heart is a chasm,
your life a stone tumbling down an infinite pit?
You take what you have and put it to work.
Service to others: that is your salvation.

A Mountain Doctor Muses

The most tragic
obstetrical cases
are the inaccessibles
left to God and nature,
the mother struggling,
straining in a cabin
back of the beyond.

Of course, those left
in the inexpert hands
of a granny woman
fare just slightly better.

Grannies know only
brews for "miseries,"
hog-greased hands,
boiled rags for the cord.

Only with reluctance
is a doctor called.
And he may feel
the same in going.
He could find
hemorrhage,
a hydrocephalic,
an impacted breech
—anything—
upon his arrival.

Mary Breckinridge on the Strength of Saplings

Before I went to France in 1918,
I was delayed in Washington.
Influenza everywhere and
hundreds in line at clinics.
So while I waited, I nursed and
noticed something remarkable:
Young clerks left their desks,
came forward to aid the sick,
so fearless we nagged them
to wear masks, to rest,
to protect themselves
lest they be stricken too.

In France I was astonished:
girls drove Ford camions
into war-ravaged villages,
delivered food, clothing,
brought wheat seed to farmers.
so life could begin again.

When we needed help with horses
in Kentucky, I wrote friends with
daughters who rode, and they came.
From Sewickly, Louisville, Shaker,
they came, paid their own way,
labored without pay, even bought
their own uniforms.
They taught new riders, carried
messages and supplies to clinics,
poulticed horses' wounds.
If needed they accompanied nurses
to birthings, chopped wood,
fed the children. Amazing.

Over and over I have learned:
in each new endeavor, call on
the young. They will astound you.

LOCAL WOMAN:
ON SADDLEBAG WOMEN

Some woman from other side of Kentucky
means to save us from our grannies.
Too much death here, she says, so she's
bringing us trained nurses, medicine. Says
they'll ride right up to the cabin to catch babies.
What I say is, ain't grannies doing that now?

We don't need no brought on women here.
Grannies know us, know whose babies
are like to step out feet first into this world.
They got warm hands, good sense. Don't need
saddlebags of supplies. Looks to me them nurses
must not know much if they need to tote stuff.

I've seen these nurses. Hard looking women.
Wear uniforms with britches, like soldiers.
I ask, what kind of woman wears trousers?
They might make it through winter,
but won't last past spring. Get some
mountain mud on those fine uniforms
and they'll be gone. You'll see.

Ain't ours to say if there's too much death.
Next thing, they'll have doctors bringing on babies.
Men! Birthing ain't no sickness, and some of us
are born just to die. That's just how it is.

Mary Breckinridge Speaks of Burdens

To birthings, our nurses carry
30-lb. saddlebags packed dense
with newspapers and rubber sheets,
aprons of rubber and cotton,
gloves, hypodermics,
a cap and gown.

They swaddle olive oil, alcohol,
Lysol in snow-clean cotton bags,
add catheters and clamps,
scissors for the umbilical,
bulb, hose of a Higginson's syringe,
basins that nestle in each other
like infants in their mothers' wombs.

They carry responsibilities
for all their patients and
the weight of their experience.

Our nurses carry their worries
about news from home
in England, Ireland, Scotland.

Even raw bone weary, they carry
themselves erect in the saddle.

They carry my expectations and
their standards for themselves,
memory maps of the way there,
nicknames—Texas, Freddie,
Mac—bestowed by fellow nurses.

Across the creek, down the mountain,
they carry gratitude for happy outcomes.

And the horses
    Dixie

Tramp
　　　Remus
　　　Beauty
　　　Raven
　　　Lady Jane
　　　Baldy Dude
　　　Nellie Gray
　　　and Rick
carry them.

Thus Sayeth the Expert: Dr. Josiah M. Slemons Weighs In on the Curse of Eve

All mammals suffer in childbirth. Anyone who observes
quadrupeds prepare for delivery knows this fact.
Their period of pain is shorter, true, because man's
upright posture has reshaped the human pelvis,
so woman's confinement is less pleasant than a cat's.
To those who inquire what purpose is served by pain,
I urge a moment's reflection. Discomfort—nature's
compelling call—is the alert that birth will soon occur.
Without such warning, the mother might be delivered
in awkward circumstances—at the theater, perhaps,
while riding a streetcar—and the infant could perish
the instant it draws breath. I simply cannot believe,
however, that suffering is essential to mother's love.
Is gold or silver that's easily gained valued any less
than what's acquired through harder purchase?

Local Woman:
Knots

Didn't I see Callie Young on her porch last week mending?
Didn't I say she ought not tie threads herself? Now
that baby is tangled, I hear, and the poor girl's suffering.

Preacher binds us, woman to man, with law and promise.
Come birthing though, it's time to loosen. Open the gate,
pull wide drawers, raise windows, unlace every shoe.

Whatever needs to run must run. You can't block
what wants to flow. That nurse can't know,
so you be my legs and go speak for our old ways.

Before you catch sight of the cabin, unpin your hair.
If an axe is in the stump, you best wrench it out.
And don't let Callie's mama clasp her hands.

I did all this for you, Hazel, when you were fast
in your mama's womb, then come to find your daddy
cross-legged in the next room the whole time.

Once he went round, whacked the beams
like God himself shaking the world right, why
you slipped out, straight into my arms.

That nurse don't know. She'll cross Big Creek
three, four times to get to Callie's place,
and then you'll have lots of straightening to do.

Lady Helen MacKenzie: Scotland Comes to Kentucky

I.

At the restaurant in the Combs Hotel
I eat enough for three hungry men.
Like a pair of maharajas, Leslie and I
perch atop a buckboard.
Then our caravan—five wagons,
innumerable riders—leaves Hazard.
The grey skies, the rocking wagon—
I could drowse all the way to Hyden.
And then the rain begins.

II.

June, cold as an Edinburgh winter.
We huddle under a tarpaulin.
Rain pours down through leaves,
onto us, the ground, mud, mud, mud.
Jonah shouts commands, urging
his mules forward (sometimes up,
sometimes down the narrow road.)
Long, low grumble of thunder,
chatter from the wagon behind us
(The Perry County Miners' Band,)
Remarkable country, Leslie murmurs.

The rain will not stop.

But Leslie dedicates the hospital
tomorrow. We must press on.

We make creeping progress,
despite wheels mired in mud.
We lessen the load, climb down,
wait in shoe-sucking mud as
Jonah prods and mules pull.

Then it's up again on the wagon
until further down (or up)
the slippery trail when the
process requires repeating.

And the rain it will not stop.

III.

Before our trip Mary told us
of Roderick McIntosh,
early settler in the area,
Highlander like ourselves.
Along the way I think of him
leaving Scotland for Virginia,
then turning his back on Virginia
for a new home, a cabin by the
creek that bears his name.

Unwavering as any Highlander
should be, he lived to be 104,
drank peach brandy each day.
I imagine him, finding his way
to Kentucky in rain and mud.

Next time I climb down,
wait in the mud, a woman shouts
I'm knee-deep in McIntosh Country.
Leslie laughs. It's me.

IV.

Tis a wee bit damp, a voice behind
mocks a brogue in our direction.
A musician, I suspect.
Leslie turns to converse
with the band, and soon we
are singing "Farewell to Tarwathie,"
sad and solemn, then, with vigor,
"Charlie is My Darlin'."
Suddenly we arrive in Hyden
bedraggled in appearance but
mid-chorus of "Raggle Taggle Gypsy,"
lusty as old friends.
As Mary greets us, there's gunfire,

a surprising welcome from Hyden's
enthused citizenry.
Within minutes the sky clears,
and then the rain,
the blessed rain, stops at last.

Mary takes us to Wendover where
the county's only bathtub awaits.
Tomorrow night, after the speeches,
there'll be a proper celebration:
roman candles and skyrockets
will brighten the night.

Watch faces, Mary tells us.
They've not seen fireworks,
So watch the children's faces.

THUS SAYETH THE EXPERT:
DR. DeLee CALLS FOR THE END TO MIDWIFERY

Childbirth is a natural process, it's true,
but it's also pathologic, often harming
mother and child. I sometimes wonder
if Nature intended that women be used
up in reproduction, like salmon who die
after spawning.

What's needed for safe deliveries is a
series of interventions—sedatives and
ether, followed by episiotomies, then
forceps—all wielded by the obstetrician.
Though disdained, obstetrics is high art.
The midwife, however, is a relic
of barbarism.

> *If an uneducated woman of the lowest classes*
> *can practice obstetrics, why, it must require*
> *very little in the way of skill and knowledge.*

That's what the public must think if
we continue to allow ignorant women
to practice our delicate profession.
No wonder young physicians
won't choose obstetrics.
How can they expect respect and
remuneration if anyone—
a neighbor, a passerby—
is thought capable?

These days even the poor foreigner,
crowded in city tenements,
is enlightened to the value of
a physician's attendance and demands it.
As for rural areas, why, midwives
are almost gone from rural Illinois.

If before this week ends, midwives across America simply vanished, women would be cared for better than before. I am certain of it.

Gwen's Highland Farewell

You'll miss Inverness, he said,
pine for your Ma and us all.

They've got horses, I answered,
and they'll teach me to ride.

Aye, there's saddlebags to carry,
forty pounds each so they say.

There's babies that need me.
Bairns are born everywhere.

The way they talk, Dad.
"On the edge of the dark."

That's poetry, that is.
Robbie Burns said it better.

You'll be among strangers.
But those hills look like home.

Moonshiners and feuders
They call us animals, scum.

Your mind is made up then?
You'll go off to Kentucky?

I was seeing myself atop
a mare in the gloaming.

You'll miss Scotland, he said,
but I had nothing to answer.

Gwen's Journey to Lenore

I. Travel

Gwen rides the train that labors up hills,
pulls across a vista of sun-struck mountains.
She has thirsted ever since the crossing.
Gwen leaves the certainty of clean sheets, adventure
administered in nightly doses of *Wuthering Heights*.
She fingers a talisman in her pocket, a glint of smoky quartz,
from Cairngorm, her father's gift. Mother only spat,
> *Take your temper with you, foolish girl.*
Stepping out at Hazard, Gwen waits for the promise
of a horse and guide to lead her over forty miles of trail.
Perhaps there will be a dog as well.

II. Arrive

Somewhere between Hazard and Hyden, Gwen adopts
her middle name. She can't resist the elegant L, its loops at top
and bottom, the way it curls upon itself like the necks of swans.
She wants to know the names of birds she sees,
wants to memorize their songs. She wants to be tempered
by the absence of inevitabilities.
> *I will be who I am to become.*
After fording Cutshin Creek, she pauses to adjust the reins, turns
in her saddle, and drops on the trail a stone the color of Scottish skies.

KATE MEDITATES ON HILLS LIKE DOMED TEMPLES

Mist curls into hollows, sinks into gaps,
cotton batting tucked up to the chin
of the mountain's darker side. *That's just Indians,*
Father's voice says. *Smoke from their teepees.*

They're cooking dinner.

I come from gridded streets, fathom my way
to any address. No signs here, no roads. Just
creek beds, deer crossings. *Take the trail cut
back of Monroe's, watch for pine on your left.*

I never get lost.

It seems I know these soft mountains,
though no one showed them to me before.
They have found me, or I have found them.
Why else should father speak so in my head?

A Memo From Mary Breckinridge: This is to Inform You That

We have thirty-seven horses and none to spare.
New riders must learn to saddle, bridle, girth
their horses. Ask experienced riders how best
to sit in the saddle without pounding the horse.
Never put on a horse any saddle but his own.
Cleanse all abrasions both noon and night.
A horse sent off duty thanks to a careless rider
costs us one dollar a day. Bad backs
on our horses are as inexcusable as mix-ups
in medications, as bedsores in the hospital.

If you injure your horse, we will assign you
the poorest ride until you learn otherwise.

LENORE GRUMBLES ABOUT UNIFORMITY

Like little colonels of the Confederacy,
we are curveless in blue-grey jackets.

Tailor made, Mrs. B says.

Breckinridge-made, more like, in her image
and woe to she whose tie slips cattywampus.

So how does she get away with it, Ireland's
Miss Priss, her red-curled flag unfurled?

Oh, I don't care for hats, says she.

The rest of us clamp down our caps, but she—
oh, too many miles today have made me sour.

Thus Sayeth the Expert:
Nurse Scovil Speaks to Prospective Mothers

We cannot take even the shortest journey
without imperiling lives. To dwell on accidents
that may never happen is as foolish as fretting
away the pleasures of an ocean voyage.

Instead, dwell on pretty pictures—mountain lakes
in summer, a forest wrapped in winter blankets,
the babe you will soon embrace—keep the ideal
before your imagination at all times.

Attend concerts or the theatre (properly dressed.)
Occupy leisure moments with literature, attend
to house plants or other agreeable diversions.
Think nothing unpleasant about the ordeal

through which you must pass. Put whatever
excites unpleasant emotion far, far away.
The crown of womanhood is at hand and soon
you will ascend to full possession of your kingdom.

Section Two

Take Root

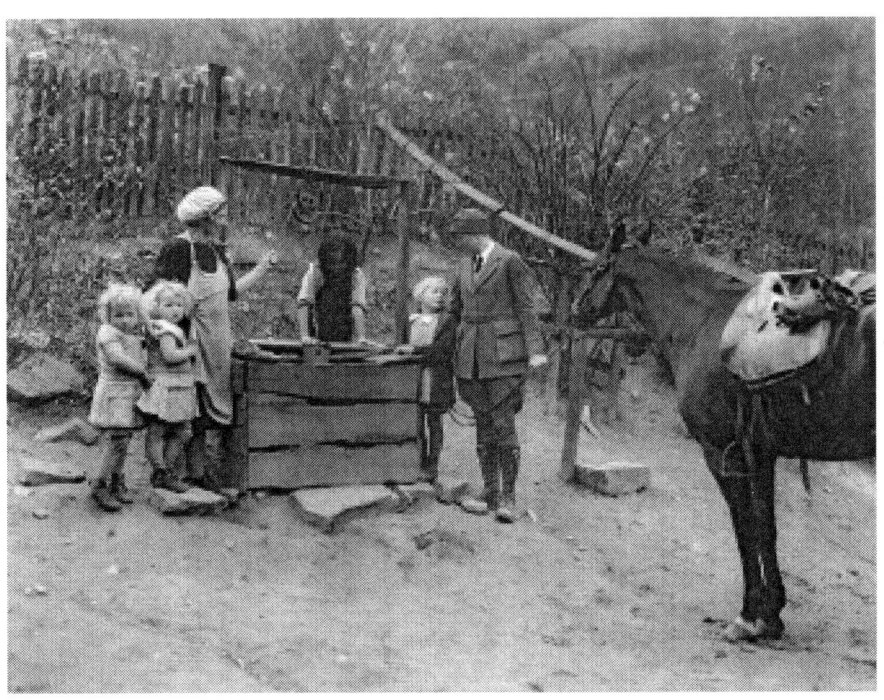

Nurse by well, 1932
(Courtesy of University of Louisville)

Mary Breckinridge Explains Mountain Medicine

One thing leads to another:
a cold becomes "brow skeeters,"
then pneumonia, perhaps death.
We see whooping cough and measles,
tonsillitis, influenza, diphtheria,
typhoid, tuberculosis, dysentery,
hookworm, hookworm, hookworm.
And calamities: deep gashes from cutting
timber, snake bites, gunshot wounds,
men crushed in their own small mines,
a girl twirling in her dress by the hearth,
burned, twin baby boys orphaned,
malnourished, like meat drying on bone.

But joys too: the twins hearty, adopted,
girls in overalls like their brothers,
netting over cribs in summer, children
lining up, waiting for vaccinations,
infected tonsils removed, bodies mended.
Some battles end up wins for our side.

Kate Sees a Haint

Stories of spirits, forced partings
of hapless lovers, the unsettled dead.
Lenore and I sat up, swapping tales
until the dogs barked. Barking means
babies, means a father has come for a nurse.
I dressed and went with him.
A first baby. The mother labored all night,
through the next day. By the time baby came
it was night again, later still before I left.
Riding home in the dark, near asleep in the saddle,
I saw something in the woods.

I passed through hemlocks, on into the oaks
when a possum bustled in the bush. No,
much larger and upright. The lantern lit on
flesh, bare arms and legs. A man it looked like,
with bark and branches where his torso should be,
and leaves around a puckish smile.
I stopped. So did he.
Dixie crunched a twig just then,
loud in all that quiet. And he left,
this man, or tree, or bit of both.
I know I saw something.

LAY OF THE LAND:
SARAH'S STALL MUCKING SONG

Bad Creek and Beech Creek, Bull Creek and Bowens,
Big Bullskin, plain Big—and that's just the Bs.
Cutshin and Elkhorn, Goose, Hector and Hell
(which Mamie insists is called Heck),
Leatherwood and Jacobs, (Lower Jacobs, that is).
Muncies and Rockhouse, Stinnett Creek—that's the last.
Something called Greasy, what it is I don't know,
but don't forget Hurricane, Hals Fork and the rivers:
Red Bird and North Fork, South Fork and Middle.

No wonder I dream of Big Bad Geese going to Hell.

"Learn them by Tuesday," Mrs. B said at tea.
"New couriers will not assist nurses til then.
Mothers and babies need our assistance, so we'll
waste no time in search of girls too lazy to learn."

No wonder I dream of Big Bad Geese going to Hell.

At home it's easy finding Father's bank and my school.
There's a sign at each corner, no chance to get lost.
But here it's rocks, creeks and mountains,
lots of trees and some cabins that all look the same.

No wonder I dream of Big Bad Geese going to Hell.

Annie, 7, Skips To The Clinic

Nurse says it's ten cents for the needles.
I have five pennies and three eggs so
I'll sweep the clinic floor for the rest
and have my own to take home.

Will they be sharp?

I'm to learn to knit on Tuesday afternoons.
If I had a sister, she'd come to Flat Creek too,
but I'd try to fool her playing Simon Says
the whole way there and back.

Simon Says hop on one foot.

From here to the clinic ain't all that far and
I'm not afraid to go there by myself.
Nurse says she will teach us knit and purl.
We will make sweaters. I want red. Or yellow.

If I had a sister I would call her Pearl.

Mama says she won't hardly stand it if they
lose this one too. They don't know I heard.
We should make blankets instead, and I'd
make one for Pearl. An orange one. Or red.

Simon Says take three steps backwards.

Horse Trading:
Sales Pitch

Western Union, Night Letter
Rec'd via Krypton, Sept. 17, 1932

Miss Mary Beckinridge
Wendover, Kentucky

    Sure have a lovely looking plantation saddle horse to please you. She is six years old, sound, fawn color, mane and tail hazel, brown eyes, good eyes, good horse, never saw a better one. Very intelligent, beautiful mare. Smooth all over, no rough points, in splendid condition. A real plantation walking mare, will run and walk and canter; won't trot under saddle. Been used on a large farm and I tested her within thirty feet of steam engine, fearless. Has spirit but sense. Sired by Marshal McDonald, great sire of walking horses; her dam is fawn colored mare, best walking mare I know. Won't you meet me in Hazard? Please answer by wire today.

C.L. Campbell

Sarah Explains Mountain Etiquette

Don't knock on a cabin door.
Wait at the fence instead.
A dog or two will bark
your arrival, but if not,
hallo the house and wait.
Some say this advice is
leftover from feuding days,
but knocking is pushy.
Why should someone jump
just because you showed up?

Oh, and turn down offers
of anything but coffee or water.
Mountaineers are generous.
They will offer food they have
little enough of for themselves.
If it's late and you're asked
to *take a night*, say no or
someone will sleep on the floor.
It won't be you.

Mary Breckinridge Calls for Stories

This is to remind you we get no government funding.
Many families can't pay our small fees, so they hew
our firewood, share their gardens' bounties.
But fathers' labors cannot equip clinics, feed horses
or supply your salaries. I've asked you for accounts
of noteworthy experiences, but received only two.
How can our generous benefactors see what we do,
understand why it matters, if we fail to enlighten them?

I can count births and babies, can compile statistics,
but you bring life to numbers, make them add up.
It's you who navigate trails, enter far-flung cabins,
see people as they are. We ask a lot of you as nurses.
We need you to tell stories. Send anecdotes soon, please.

Nancy Tries To Tell It

I'm no writer, I tell Mrs. B.
"Just tell it," she says. Nothing fancy is required."
So here it is:

There is a rule here. If the father can get to us,
we are obliged to accompany him. No matter
what the weather nor how far the cabin,
we must go. Mountain travel is arduous,
especially in early Spring when—

No, no, try again, Nancy. How would you tell this
to your own sweet mother back in Ireland?

Flood smashed through the other night
with water enough to jolt Jesus himself.
A man came for me around nine o'clock.
Path washed out behind him, we took
the long way round, a most terrible trail
indeed. Paddy and I saw Hurricane Creek
four times; the father struggled in water
rushing and roaring up to his neck.

Pleasant fellow, this father, but he's no
Finn MacCumhail. He'll throw out no stones,
construct no causeway to keep our feet dry.

Near midnight another storm began
as we arrived. Wind rushed like Satan
between chinks in the walls, gaps in the floor.
And light from the coal lamp nearly danced
to death. But the young mother was calm,
thank heavens. I kept my coat on and caught
an 11-lb. baby at two. Before I left, mother
and babe were tucked up, asleep. The father?
He grinned and grinned and grinned.

I crossed the clinic's threshold at seven
and tumbled myself into bed.

Sarah's Letter Home:
Tower to Tank and Across the Creek

April 12, 1932

Dear Mother,

Remember that summer in Atlantic City?
How we children begged each day for a trip
to the Steel Pier. Gerald so certain he'd win
games of chance, Estelle prattling on about
taffy and trinkets. And me, desperate to see
Sonora and the High Diving Horse. Forty feet,
they said, from the tower to the tank.

You relented at last, and after the carousal,
sandwiches and rests in the shade—you
could have told me, Mother, about the baby
—we filed into the arena. And oh, the build up!
Hundreds of people restless in their seats.
The announcer tells how perilous the dive,
how courageous horse and rider, and then hush.
Sonora appears atop the platform, her horse
gallops the long slow ramp. A baby or a
seagull cries, I hear the ocean hum, and all
those people are silent. Suddenly, all around me
a great cry. I open my eyes and watch Sonora
and her horse swim to the tank's edge. Such
noise then, such cheers for brave Sonora.

Spring's thaw gushes our creeks, pours water
down mountains, and rivulets become oceans.
To ford Hell-for-Sartain yesterday, I stood
in Jo's saddle and together we strained
for the shore. I tried to envision spectators
in tiers up the mountain, shading their eyes,
breathless, yet the image would not come.
My eyes though, Mother, my eyes were open.

Horse Trading:
Mary Breckinridge Returns a Horse

We are returning the horse you delivered yesterday.
He is too old. For a horse his age, your price is too high.

        We think him not much under fifteen.

We give our horses constant hard riding,
and find it impractical to buy them over ten.

Sweet feed has made him fat, an undesirable trait.
We cannot keep an unprofitable horse that long.

        We will send him back early next week.

If you get hold of two good saddlers—young, gentle—
in fair condition, we assure you they will be purchased.

Kate's Lament

I went to Wendover to care for the horses;
I stayed for two years instead of three months.

My mother sent me to work with the horses,
to help the nurses traverse the dense hills.

I stayed for the laurel, the mothers, the babies;
I stayed for the horses: for Paddy and Bear.

For tea at Wendover and lunch with Miss Mary,
for laughter at midnight and my dear Diane.

I'd stay for forever if Diane wouldn't marry,
I'd stay and slop stalls for Paddy and Bear.

But I read her betrothal in a paper from Richmond
on the wall of a cabin round the mountain past Hell.

I helped the nurse with another hard birthing,
then stood in the snow while the horses breathed frost.

I'm leaving Wendover, going back to the city;
please tell her I said goodbye to the horses and all.

Sarah's Journal: Keening

June 1, 1932

Expect blood, Lenore said.
Less than I thought but bolder,
brighter than imagined,

such a fluid jewel.
*More than one's named Ruby
in remembrance.*

But she didn't warn about
the mother's moaning.
Keening, she called it.

A low, endless mourning,
like a beast snared under the bed,
deep, deep and seeping out,

up through weary floorboards
from far below the cabin
and somewhere lower still.

An underworld lament
coiled past arrowheads
older than the Cherokee,

a stubborn seedling,
music pressed fern-like
into rock, it emerged

finally, as a new song.
Then: a baby cried and
the mother laughed.

Horse Trading:
Mary Keeps a Horse

We like your mare and are disposed to keep her.
You say Daisy is a fine saddle horse, easy on a rider,
but may we have a statement from you declaring
she is not in foal? She is fat and we cannot be sure.

If you send us a guarantee that she is not expecting,
agreeing to take her back and return our money
in case she is, we will keep her and send a check
in payment for Daisy and her equipment ($125).

Sarah's Letter Home:
A Cabin in Arles

June 19, 1932

Mother, remember the museum
and the painting we admired?
Van Gogh's bed and chair in France,
his snug little bedroom
shimmering in blues and orange?
I went into a cabin today
just as small.
La Chambre a' Arles worked
in down-to-earth brown
here in Kentucky.

The husband was off timbering,
the mother there alone with
her first child, a girl in brown hair,
handmade dress. Heavy as she
was, she lumbered
out of bed to make a kind of tea.
Smelled like a summer forest,
bits of plant floating,
like a creek after a storm.
I sipped politely.

The mother—barely my age—
her child already four,
living in a room bare except for
bed and table, chairs,
a kettle over the fire.
Instead of pictures,
newspaper pasted across walls,
a room blank as a cave.

I toyed with my tea, watched Laura,
who shied like a pony at first.

She twirled and sang to her doll,
then demanded a story as
Lenore consulted the mother.

I don't know what my face said but
as we rode home,
Lenore turned in the saddle,
>*Just because they have nothing
doesn't mean they are nothing.*

I will do better next time, but Mother,
those chairs, imagine, beautifully
caned just like Van Gogh's.

HORSE TRADING:
GIFT HORSE

Mr. William Kerr to Mrs. Mary Breckinridge

> I sold to W.M. Monroe today a beautiful black mare,
> six years old, named Annette. Gentle saddle horse.
> He is making you a present of it. I want to ship tomorrow.
> Wire back today about where I may send her. Would you
> see about getting me a railroad discount since this mare
> is for your frontier service and the nurses?

Mrs. Mary Breckinridge to Mr. William Kerr

> I am sure Annette is a nice horse but do not ship her here.
> We work in rough country, almost no ground on which
> a horse can canter. We carry heavy saddlebags filled
> with bottles for care of the sick and have no use for
> horses that trot. Our horses need a fast running walk
> as well as reasonably fast flat-footed walk. The trot
> breaks our bottles, the canter is impossible. Many
> thanks for your care selecting what will no doubt be
> a delightful saddle mare for hunting around Lexington.

Kate's Case of Mountainitus

Sewickley, Penn.
Oct. 12, 1932

Friends,

Since my return to Pennsylvania
I have contracted a grave disease.
Prognosis for this patient is poor.
Unless a remedy is administered,
she will collapse and commence
clucking like a chicken, neighing
like a horse, jabbering about tea.
Under doctor's orders, I will arrive
in Hazard next Monday.

Will one of you meet me at the station?

Kate

Sarah's Journal:
Fecundity

July 23, 1932

Insects rage tonight,
frenetic noise.
Locusts and I don't know what else.
I'm accustomed to Marie's snores,
but frenzy won't let me sleep—
the woods a tuning orchestra
and I have fallen into the pit.
Never just one or two of anything here
but life by the dozens,
uncountable multitudes
of bugs, trees, birds, plants.

I have seen only one
luna moth,
luminous green,
large as my hand.
Lucas pitied me when I asked what it was.
Deems my life impoverished,
I who must ask
so many questions.
The moth was dying.
Eager ants fed on its body
as legs pedaled still.
They only live a week, Lucas said
but I doubted and took down
the Britannica.
He was right.
Their sole purpose is to mate,
not even a mouth for feeding.
Their eggs become caterpillars, pupa, then moths
on and on, life in a cycle and so brief.

Yesterday at the Morgan's I waited outside
with horses and children while Lenore visited

mother and babe. Saw a sapling growing
out from under the cabin,
leaning, twisting to reach the sun.
Perhaps wind blew a seed there or
a bird dropped one
through the porch boards.
Such an unsound place to begin life.
Made me think of May when
it looked like snow had come
to Beech Fork, whirling at our feet,
clumping by the barn.
Just fuzzies, Lucas said,
floating down from cottonwoods
that line the river,
their seed a small passenger.

Such a will in living things to start anew.

When you are alone by Mrs. B's fireplace
and brush your fingers across
the brass plaque

> *To the Glory of God*
> *and in memory of*
> *Breckie and Polly Breckinridge*
> *Dedicated Christmas 1925*

you see how this all began with death and
a resolve to start again.

Section Three

Grow

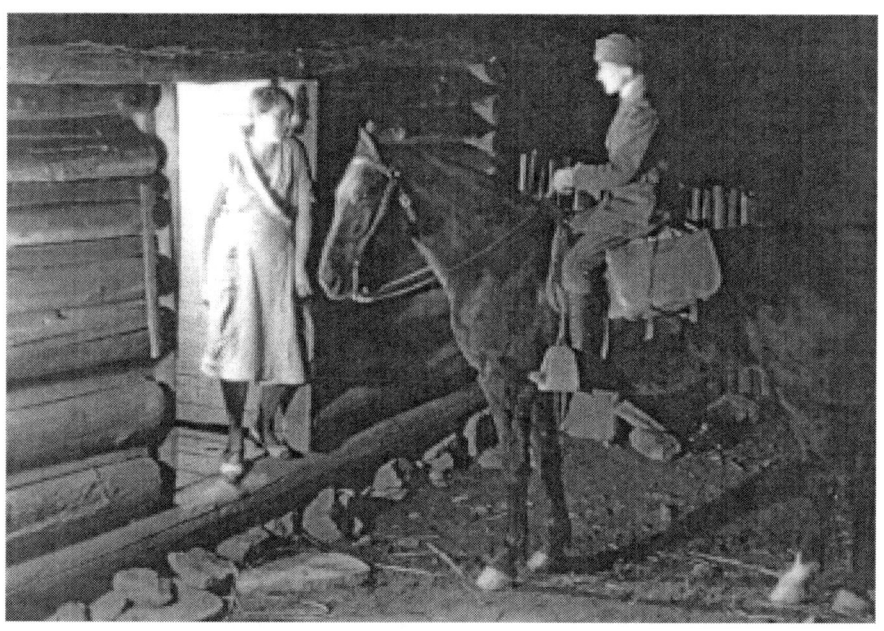

Nurse visiting woman in cabin at night c. 1932.
(Courtesy of FNU)

Frontier Nursing Service Bulletin: Will You Fill Their Saddlebags?

They're riding today on America's frontier.
Up overgrown trails, across rushing rivers
on their way to save a life, perhaps two.
It could be Marcus, a boy with a fever,
little Sally with a broken arm, or Helen,
a young mother facing her agony
in a lonesome cabin. Their lives depend
on nurses and the saddlebags you fill.

Frontier nurses ride horseback
through Kentucky's roughest country
where roads are mere bridle trails,
streams are seldom bridged,
automobiles never find their way.
Send a dollar to buy their horses feed,
ten dollars to deliver a newborn safely
into a mother's arms. Don't delay.

Send a check to the Frontier Nursing Service.

Hyden Man Peruses Sunday Paper

Reading the rotogravure,
pages the color of tea and
Meemaw's oldest linens,
I see a photograph of
our bank and Eversole store.
The picture snapped just as
four pigs sashay down the street.

I'm not saying there's never
been livestock in town, but
city papers are mighty good
at noting any rickety cabin or
toothless granny around here.
They want people to pity
"poor, ignorant mountain folk."
No wonder city people believe
Kentucky is full to the brim with
lifeless results of blood feuds,
winsome mountain girls,
'shiners passing the jug.

Pity the poor mountain folk?
Hear this: We are not ignorant.
We do not need pity.
And couldn't you have waited
for the pigs to pass?

Annie, 9, Takes a Stand

Doctor coming from Louisville
to take your tonsils, Momma says.
Don't you act up none, don't you fuss.

Nurse says, *He'll have long shiny tools,*
it will be snip, snip over in a second
and then there will be ice cream.

Never had my tonsils out before
but ice cream's nothing new.
I won't leave Momma and Daddy,
won't climb up on the wagon,
ride with all those other children.

Nurse says, *Hospital beds are full up*
but there will be a pallet on the floor,
other children and lots of ice cream,
as much as you could ever want.

She must think me a fool.

The Moon Man Speaks

Preacher come last week, started on
about miracles, about Jesus and ten lepers.
Preacher, I told him, *this old tree I'm in
can't hold more than five sick fellows.*
Not so much as a smile from him,
but when he bowed his head,
and I saw that bald spot—
I about laughed myself sick.
He ain't been back since.

Miz Neville from other side of Bowens
come by too. I heard her a long way off,
scratching her way up the trail,
panting like a hound in August.
Held an elderberry pie up so high I could smell it.
Save it for the wake nearly slipped out,
but what I said was *thank you, ma'am.*
Children ate the pie.

Wendover nurse was here,
hands on her hips like a soldier.
Looked hot from that uniform,
but red-faced, mad hot, too.
Blamed Dixon for putting me up this tree.
Took all I had in me to holler down.
Soon as I knew it was the lung disease,
I asked Dixon and his boy to build a pallet
and up I climbed. So I'm near enough to see
my kin but far enough not to harm.
'Sides, Dixon asked her, *what can
some hospital do that his people can't?*

Dixon's boy brings me food, water,
dumps my pot down the privy.
Mary washes the rags I cough in,
and the little girls scamper out
the cabin, sing me songs, ask for stories.
They grin up at me, those little faces,

* * *

I figure I must look far away
as the man in the moon.
Make a wish on me, I tell them.
Your Uncle Hense will make it true.
Nurse says she'll come back here,
thinks a passel of men could lift me
out, thinks she can make me well too.
My coming down will be harder
than the going up, she'll see.

Smells good up here.
Cabin fire, wet earth when it rains.
Thought it might rain some last night
when a little breeze come through,
made leaves sway and chatter
like biddies before church.

I don't see sky though—trees so full
it's always near dark in this hollow.
Come autumn and I'm still here, leaves
will float down, and I'll see clouds then.

Nancy and the Moon Man

Somebody round here sick?

A voice familiar
but I could not recall
a face. How could I?
Large eyes, big enough
to slice open darkness;
a graybone man,
peering through a confusion
of chestnut leaves,
right down to the ground
right down to me.

Well, if it ain't that red-haired nurse.

Mrs. Neville told me about him,
said he'd moved from cabin
to tree some time before Easter.
Thought he had "the lung disease";
Oh, he does, he does, I know it,
she said.

When the axe slipped when
Meryl Parker's boy cut timber
in the woods, I cleaned the wound,
called for a stretcher and one appeared.
He'd made it: saplings passed
through coats; green saplings
like long, delicate bones jutting out
the red plaid sleeves. Mountaineers
watched me fumble through my
ministrations. No one shivered
but me and the boy.

When I stood at the back
of the church while Brownie
explained why bleach
must be poured down

all the mountain's wells,
a man nudged and whispered,

    What's this about a German theory?

Germ. I said, *Germ,*
not German. Glanced up
into a grin and it was his.
Back then I thought stupid
and uneducated were the same.

Climbing up from the river,
thumb on Mrs. Neville's map,
I hoped to find only pneumonia,
or whooping cough or
something else.

And now I know him:
Hense Morgan,
late of this hollow,
son of Richard and
Naomi (deceased,)
brother of Dixon and
Mary, beloved uncle
to five Morgan children.

We will somehow
carry him down.

Miss Marvin Makes a Movie: Marvin in the River

Up to my shins in I'm-forgetting-which river,
    (crank, crank, crank)
turning the Kodak's stiff handle.
    (crank, crank, crank)
Mary says film it, I ask when and where,
    (crank, crank, crank)
keeping the rhythm with hands that are numb.
    (crank, crank, crank)
"Spring" Mary calls it but surely it's winter.
    (crank, crank, crank)
Do it again I call out and the volunteers groan.
    (crank, crank, crank)
Once more and then tea, I foolishly promise, but
    (crank, crank, crank)
get the stroke wrong and the film's underexposed.
    (crank, crank, crank)
If only, if only I knew how to do this,
    (crank, crank, crank)
I'd make Mary proud and a movie besides.
    (crank, crank, crank)

LENORE AT THE BRINK

Crossing rivers unnerves me still,
and here it is Spring with nothing
but rain. The creek is ever rising.
At its worst, Tramp and I swim,
each muscle in his body at war
against a rage of moving water.

Every time we ford Big Creek
Jenny Greenteeth comes to mind
and I stop at the edge.
From the dust of my childhood
she emerges, flashes her fangs.
Get too close to the river, she'll
sing *Come into the water, love.*
She'll reach out, arms stretching,
long hair swirling, whirling,
her bony fingers grasping.
She'll pull you in, drag you down,
snare you in duckweed 'til you drown.

Even worse than Jenny is the kelpie,
shape-shifting demon in his
white horse disguise. He'll whisper
Come ride with me, love.
But once you climb on he leaves
land, plunges into deep water,
looks back to watch you perish.

But at river's edge, I remember:
Jenny never was, Tramp's no kelpie.
I say a quick prayer and we step in.

NANCY DESCRIBES THE TOPOGRAPHY

To find McBurney's Point,
draw a line from your navel
to iliac crest, the highest part
of your pelvic bone. Then
trace fingers two thirds down
that line. Press.
If condition is acute, you will howl.

To find your way from Wendover
to Cutshin Clinic, head east.
Cross Wolf Creek, pass the cabin
where I made my last call, ascend
to the meadow where I studied stars.
From there you can see down
to clinic and barn.

To get from hospital to motor road,
line up behind men taking
turns with my coffin.
Step in behind mourners and Raven,
stirrups crossing an empty saddle.
We'll pick our way down
the winding path from there.

Mary Breckinridge Contemplates One Bright Star

At the funeral we sang
> *O Valiant hearts who*
> *to your glory came*
> *through dust of conflict*
> *and through battle flame.*

That's a war hymn, someone said.
We are at war, I thought
though I was too tired to say it.
At war with disease, our failures.

I want to forget:
the poison's slow assault
a too-late surgery,
our desperate nursing
gone for naught.

I hope to remember:
Nancy on her deathbed
naming her patients,
one and then another,
and then another still,
telling which
need our visit, our care.
As if dying were temporary,
a shopping trip to Lexington,
coltsfoot abloom on the trail.

> *Your memory hallowed*
> *in the land you love*
> *like some bright star*

We buried her near my children,
chiseled *Valiant Heart* on her stone.
Just the one heart.

LENORE ENCOUNTERS POETRY

She's pretty as a poem, I remarked
and in the next second Ninnie Hillman
named her newborn baby that: Poem.

I tried to talk her out of it, suggested
she take some time to think it over,
but she raised up her chin just so
and that was that.

I like the feel of it in my mouth, she said,
the little puff of air you make to say it.
Ain't no one else named such a thing
so she will be her own self in this world.

I wondered what she knew of poetry
and as if she read my mind she said,
Words of ballads, they're poems.
I grew up hearing all of those.
Daddy knows "Casey at the Bat"
and will say it start to end if you ask.
And "The Shooting of Dan McGrew."
Daddy'll be tickled with the baby's name.

"She walks in beauty like the night."
I remember that from school.
That'll be my girl when she's grown,
out walking in the night,
stars sparkling through the trees.
She'll be just as pretty as a poem.

Rose: Dead Tired

Granny Whitcomb says she can't help me. (*Can't?* snorts Tom. *Won't, more like.*) She's been catching babies for forty years now. She did for my mama and Tom's, and was here for nearly every baby born on this mountain. Now she says no, no more. Tom is mad, thinking she's stubborn. Says old people are like that but that she will come round.

I clambered up to her place one cool afternoon. Rhododendrons blooming along the way, pink blossoms peeking from under the leaves like fairies in a story, and me feeling like a bride going up a long church aisle to her true wedding. But Granny Whitcomb turned away. Offered me a drink of water, called me "child," but didn't invite me to sit. (*That's alright. Babies can get born just fine without that old woman,* Tom says.)

Granny handed me the cup, dried her hands on her apron, and said *No, no more babies* and turned away. Said *You'd better get back on home before dark.* Then Mama came to me when I was asleep, wringing her hands and saying, *I'm not sick. Just tired.* Woke up thinking maybe Granny won't be here when it's my time, and no one is coming up behind her.

And now I feel like I'm coming home in the dark wood, the rhododendron blossoms brown, the path overgrown and gone. I am alone in a moonless night. Who will help me if I lose my way?

Tom's Vow

My wife Rose says she will have herself a nurse if she has to walk to Wendover herself, but I ain't sure. Mama says she had Granny Whitcomb for all her babies and ain't we breathing still?

Maybe she forgot my sister Jane lost a baby, but I remember. I was shorter than a calf back then and not much older. It was winter but they sent me out to the barn cause Jane was suffering with that baby, and Granny Whitcomb couldn't do a damn thing for her but put her blue-veined old hand against Jane's cheek and say, *It's alright, child.*

When it was over Papa come get me. When he said the baby was lost, I ran right out the cabin door, looking for tracks in the snow. Searched and searched till I couldn't go no further, and he had to come find me. Mama likes to say I was way up the mountain by then, and wasn't that sweet of me to go looking for Jane's little baby?

Rose's own mama died with a granny beside her. Child-bed fever. At the end her mama was puny as a newborn herself, Rose says. Took her two weeks to die and nobody could do nothing.

If I had my way, I'd get every last granny in Leslie County. I'd line them all up on one side of the porch, herbs and grease all ready. And then I'd get all them nurses, make them stand at alert on the other side, soldiers waiting for battle, cause this is my Rose. She should have what she wants and then some.

MARVIN MAKES A MOVIE:
THE FORGOTTEN FRONTIER

Somebody said we took the roof off a man's cabin to film the baby scene. That's not true. He had taken the old one off himself because he was preparing to put on a new one, so we took advantage and filmed in daylight inside a mountain cabin. (I had a new camera then, one with a spring. I could wind it like a clock and it ran for several minutes on its own.) Like all the actors we used, the man and his family volunteered to be in the movie. They wanted to help the nurses who were helping them, they said. No one was paid a penny. Oh, yes, some men were given lunch at the hospital in return for helping out, but no money ever changed hands.

Raven Speaks

I am trapped
between boulder   and   tree
                     on my back
working my legs
like a bug on the barn floor

can't see ground   my body

smell of blood   excrement

Sky-blinded   I thirst
in my eyes   flies writhe

              I want her to call   me
                     come for me,

  I want to stand
     at edge of river   and drink

Edge of the dark and
a hawk floats   circles
 my name wafts on the wind
        I hear them coming
              see men   gun
                       oh, Epona

SARAH SPEAKS OF NEW TROUBLES

Broken as a china teacup that slips from a soapy hand,
demolished like a bottle of oil in a dropped saddlebag,
Katie is shattered. This new calamity has sobered us all,
but my strongest friend is distraught, speaks of going home.
Nancy's Raven, has died. Somehow she slid down
an embankment in the pasture, was wedged on her back,
caught between a beech tree and a boulder. Workmen
hewed the tree, but it was too late, or the fall too great.
Katie, strong through Nancy's illness, is inconsolable.

Our horses are stalwart, not invulnerable. They trek long
hours in all weather. We must rely on one another.

Miss Marvin Makes a Movie:
An Evening of Hoopla

Despite ball-length taffeta gowns,
despite delicate high-heeled slippers,
fifteen debutantes scamper up and down
stairs of Mecca Hall for my film's premiere.
I try to picture them bedecked as they are
ascending Kentucky mountain paths, as if
my giggling could calm my anxious mind.
The girls usher our patrons to their seats
any one of whom, cousin Mary mentions,
could be our next big benefactor,
endower of a clinic or barn or both.

        What have I gotten into now?

The hall is full and the crowd buzzes
like dragonflies in August. I am nervous.
Ruth Draper will perform a monologue,
then Tertius Noble will seat himself
at the organ to play during the movie,
my movie, my sad attempt at a movie.

        Why did I agree to come tonight?

I love the city but would sooner groom
horses at Wendover than be here now.
I wish I'd filmed more scenes, edited
more capably, knew what I was doing.
If only the product equaled my vision,
if only I weren't a perfectionist, I could
stop wringing my hands and breathe.

Sarah's Letter Home: New Moon

June 3, 1933

Dear Mother,

We're having a perfect plague of babies.
This week we've had two at Confluence,
three at Beech Fork, another at Red Bird.

Here at Brutus the Spurlock twins are due.
I credit the moon.

Lenore teases, calls me *silly goose*,
but I think there's some connection.
The moon is waxing now, grows heavy.
Soon it will be a perfect circle,
splendidly round and fat and full.
Haze embraces it on muggy nights,
a halo, as if it's something sacred.

Why couldn't the moon bring babies?
Didn't ancient people worship it?
The changing moon dictates tides,
farmers plant with an eye on it.
We can't know all its mysteries.

June's is the Moon of Horses, I'm told.
Our horses whicker as it approaches
as if muttering secrets to each other—
I know that sounds so foolish.

But Mother, this is serious:
I've been charting babies and moons.
In a year I'll know if there's a connection.
I said I'd return to Brown in Autumn
but can't you see? I've a study to complete.

Mary Breckinridge Puts It in Perspective

Today at Wendover
> two interminable meetings
> the specter of deficit by year's end
> new reports of dysentery
> a mother-to-be who walked three days to find us.

Now, twilight on the mountain
> ashen moon
> deep stillness, until a breeze reshuffles the leaves
> hills of indigo and mauve,
> the rounded shoulders of a thousand sleeping babies.

EPILOGUE

Vespers at Wendover

Arrive at twilight, in-between time,
(*edge of the dark*, they call it here).
Let the terrier from up the road escort you
to the door. Mouth clichés as you enter—
it's smaller (larger) than expected.
Consume the chicken salad waiting for you,
then wander. Note Pig Alley where people
once lined for inoculations, the dining room
where couriers poured nurses their tea.
Finger-read the hearth plaque.
In Mary's room (*your* room) admire
her diploma, photos. Watch a daddy-longlegs
make his stilted amble across your pillow,
deem him a cordial omen. Raise the window,
stretch out across the bed, surrender yourself
to the clamorous insect night.

ABOUT THE WRITER

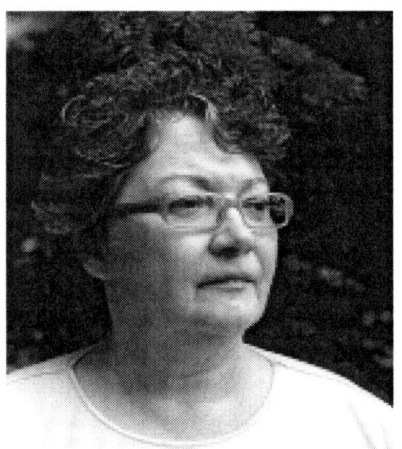

Karen Kotrba was raised in Columbiana, Ohio, where her interest in nursing history was sparked by her mother's career in nursing. An award winning writer of short fiction and essays, she graduated from the Northeast Ohio MFA program and teaches composition at Youngstown State University. She lives in Columbiana County and is currently working on a series of short stories set in East Liverpool, Ohio. Karen has led writing workshops at the Cleveland Clinic and various community settings.

Recent Books by Bottom Dog Press

Appalachian Writing Series

The Homegoing: A Novel
by Michael Olin-Hitt, 180 pgs. $18

She Who Is Like a Mare: Poems of Mary Breckinridge and the Frontier Nursing Service
by Karen Kotrba, 96 pgs. $16

Smoke: Poems
by Jeanne Bryner 96 pgs. $16

Broken Collar: A Novel
by Ron Mitchell, 234 pgs. $18

The Pattern Maker's Daughter: Poems
by Sandee Gertz Umbach, 90 pages $16

The Free Farm: A Novel
by Larry Smith, 306 pgs. $18

Sinners of Sanction County: Stories
by Charles Dodd White, 160 pgs. $17

Learning How: Stories, Yarns & Tales
by Richard Hague, 216 pgs. $18

The Long River Home: A Novel
by Larry Smith, 230 pgs. cloth $22; paper $16

Eclipse: Stories
by Jeanne Bryner 150 pgs. $16

Appalachian Anthologies

Degrees of Elevation: Short Stories of Contemporary Appalachia
Eds. Charles Dodd White and Page Seay 186 pgs. $18

Bottom Dog Press
http://smithdocs.net

RECENT BOOKS BY
BOTTOM DOG PRESS

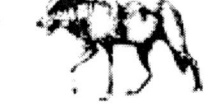

WORKING LIVES SERIES
Breathing the West: Great Basin Poems
by Liane Ellison Norman, $16
Americana Poet: a Novel
by Jeff Vande Zande, 160 pgs. $18
Selected Correspondence of Kenneth Patchen
ed. Allen Frost, cloth $28; paper $18
The Way-Back Room: Memoir of a Detroit Childhood
by Mary Minock, 216 pgs. $18
Strangers in America: A Novel
by Erika Meyers, 140 pgs. $16
Riders on the Storm: A Novel
by Susan Streeter Carpenter, 404 pgs. $18
The Long River Home by Larry Smith
230 pgs. cloth $22; paper $16
Landscape with Fragmented Figures
by Jeff Vande Zande, 232 pgs. $16
The Big Book of Daniel: Collected Poems
by Daniel Thompson, 340 pgs. cloth $22; paper $18
Reply to an Eviction Notice: Poems
by Robert Flanagan, 100 pgs. $15
An Unmistakable Shade of Red & The Obama Chronicles
by Mary E. Weems, 80 pgs. $15
d.a.levy & the mimeograph revolution
eds. Ingrid Swanberg & Larry Smith, 276 pgs. & dvd $25
Our Way of Life: Poems
by Ray McNiece, 128 pgs. $14

WORKING ANTHOLOGIES
On the Clock: Contemporary Short Stories of Work
eds. Josh Maday & Jeff Vande Zande 226 pgs. $18

BOTTOM DOG PRESS
http://smithdocs.net

CPSIA information can be obtained at www.ICGtesting.com
Printed in the USA
BVOW01s1105170314

347805BV00002B/26/P